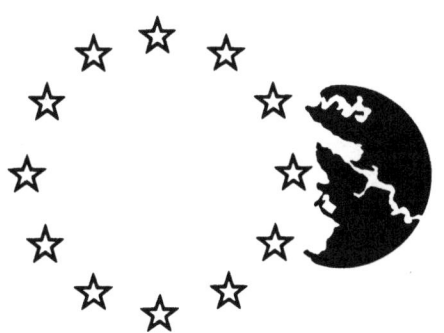

EUROPE AGAINST CANCER

European Commission Series
for General Practitioners

W0050006

Prepared for the Commission
of the European Communities
by the

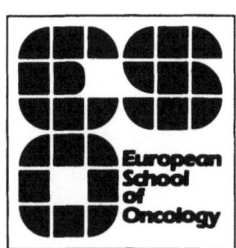

J. D. Hardcastle (Ed.)

Colorectal Cancer

Textbook for General Practitioners

Contributors
M. Crespi   M. F. Dixon   O. Kronborg   J. Wahrendorf   N. S. Williams

With 15 Figures and 2 Tables

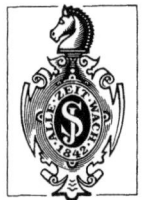

Springer-Verlag
Berlin Heidelberg New York
London Paris Tokyo
Hong Kong Barcelona
Budapest

Professor Dr. Jack Donald Hardcastle

Department of Surgery
Floor E West Block
University Hospital
Queen's Medical Centre
Nottingham NG7 2UH, UK

Warning: Neither the Commission of the European Communities nor any person acting on its behalf can accept responsibility for any use made of the information contained herein.

ISBN-13:978-3-540-56702-8   e-ISBN-13:978-3-642-78225-1
DOI:10.1007/978-3-642-78225-1

Library of Congress Cataloging-in-Publication Data
Colorectal cancer: textbook for general practitioners / J. D. Hardcastle (ed.)
   "Europe against cancer"
Includes bibliographical references.

1. Colon (Anatomy)--Cancer. 2. Rectum--Cancer. I. Hardcastle, J. D. (Jack Donald) [DNLM: 1. Colorectal Neoplasms. WI 520 C71955 1993] RC280.C6C673 1993 616.99'4347--dc20

This work is subject to copyright. All rights are reserved, whether the whole or part of the material is concerned, specifically the rights of translation, reprinting, reuse of illustrations, recitation, broadcasting, reproduction on microfilm or in any other way, and storage in data banks. Duplication of this publication or parts thereof is permitted only under the provisions of the German Copyright Law of September 9, 1965, in its current version, and permission for use must always be obtained from Springer-Verlag. Violations are liable for prosecution under the German Copyright Law.

© Springer-Verlag Berlin Heidelberg 1993

The use of general descriptive names, registered names, trademarks, etc. in this publication does not imply, even in the absence of a specific statement, that such names are exempt from the relevant protective laws and regulations and therefore free for general use.

Product liability: The publishers cannot guarantee the accuracy of any information about dosage and application contained in this book. In every individual case the user must check such information by consulting the relevant literature.

Typesetting: Data conversion by Springer-Verlag

19/3145-543210 – Printed on acid-free paper

Foreword

The "Europe against Cancer" programme has, from its inception, emphasised the key role which general practitioners must play in the actions necessary to achieve its aim of reducing the incidence and the mortality from cancer in the European Community.

General practitioners, because of their day-to-day direct and continuing contact with patients, play a role not only in primary prevention and education of patients, but also in motivating their patients to accept secondary prevention and screening, some of it carried out by general practitioners themselves. These preventive activities are in addition to their traditional role in the care and management of patients with cancer at home, and increasingly, their role in active treatment.

In view of the importance of the general practitioner in the "Europe against Cancer" programme, the European Commission, with a view to providing general practitioners with up-to-date useful information, has sponsored the production of this series of publications on organbased cancers, especially written for general practitioners.

Regis Malbois

Advisor in charge
of the "Europe against Cancer" programme
Commission of the European Communities
Brussels

Preface

Colorectal cancer is the second most common cause of death from malignant disease with a high incidence in many European countries. This book is part of a series of publications on major cancer diseases designed for the European family doctor. It is published by the Commission of the European Communities within the context of the Europe Against Cancer Programme.

This book on colorectal cancer presents, in a concise form, information that the General Practitioner needs in his day-to-day practice, with particular emphasis on aetiology, prevention, early diagnosis and screening.

The surgical management issues in colorectal cancer are discussed, together with a review of adjuvant therapy. The book has been produced by a group of experts and covers many disciplines involved in the management of colorectal cancer.

J. D. Hardcastle

Acknowledgments:
The authors would like to acknowledge the assistance of Mrs E Reavill in the production of the manuscript and Mrs G Lee in the preparation of the illustrations.

Contents

Editorial Board

Professor M. Crespi
Istituto Regina Elena per lo studio e la cura dei tumori, viale Regina Elena 291
00161 Roma, Italy

Dr. M. F. Dixon
Department of Pathology, University of Leeds, Leeds, UK

Professor O. Kronborg
Department of Surgery, Odense University, Odense, Denmark

Professor J. Wahrendorf
German Cancer Research Center, 69120 Heidelberg, Federal Republic of Germany

Professor N. S. Williams
Surgical Unit, The Royal London Hospital, Whitechapel, London, UK

We wish to acknowledge the assistance of Dr Marco Caperle in the section
"Symptoms and Investigations".

Editorial Board

How Frequent is Colorectal Cancer?

Cancers of the colon and rectum are among the most frequent causes of illness and death in Europe and in the world. There are every year in the EEC countries, about 130,000 newly diagnosed cases and about 90,000 deaths from colorectal cancer.

In the northern countries of the EEC colorectal cancer represents the second most frequent cause of death due to malignant neoplasms in both males and females, following lung cancer and breast cancer respectively. In Portugal, Spain, Italy and Greece it ranks number three.

Figure 1 gives for males and females the proportion of cancer deaths at the major sites in the Federal Republic of Germany in 1981. Colorectal cancer represents 12.3% of all cancer deaths in males and 14.8% in females.

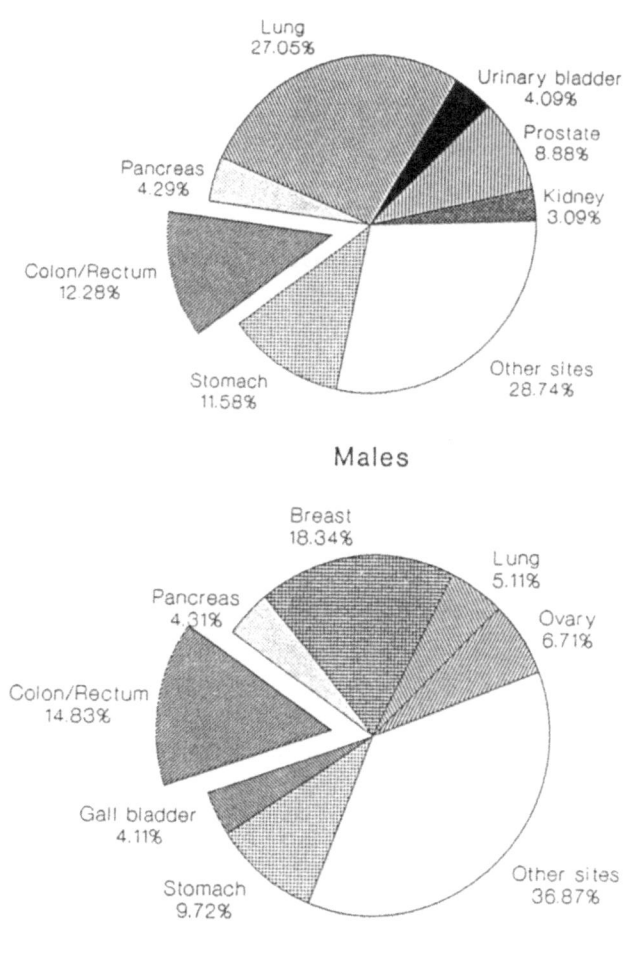

Fig. 1. Percentage of cancer deaths at major sites Federal Rebulic of Germany

1

In most European countries the male/female ratio is both for incidence and mortality in the order of 1.3. When calculated separately for colon cancer and rectum cancer, the ratio is lower (closer to one) for colon cancer and higher for rectal cancer.

Trends in Incidence and Mortality

Age-standardized mortality rates for colon cancer have remained fairly stable over the last three decades in countries where the mortality had initially been high and has shown an increase in countries with initially lower mortality. However, a slight levelling-off of this increase has been observed in recent years; indeed, moderate declines in rectal cancer mortality have been observed in several countries.

In Figure 2 age-standardized incidence rates for cancers of the intestines, chiefly colon and rectum are given for some European and non-European populations covered

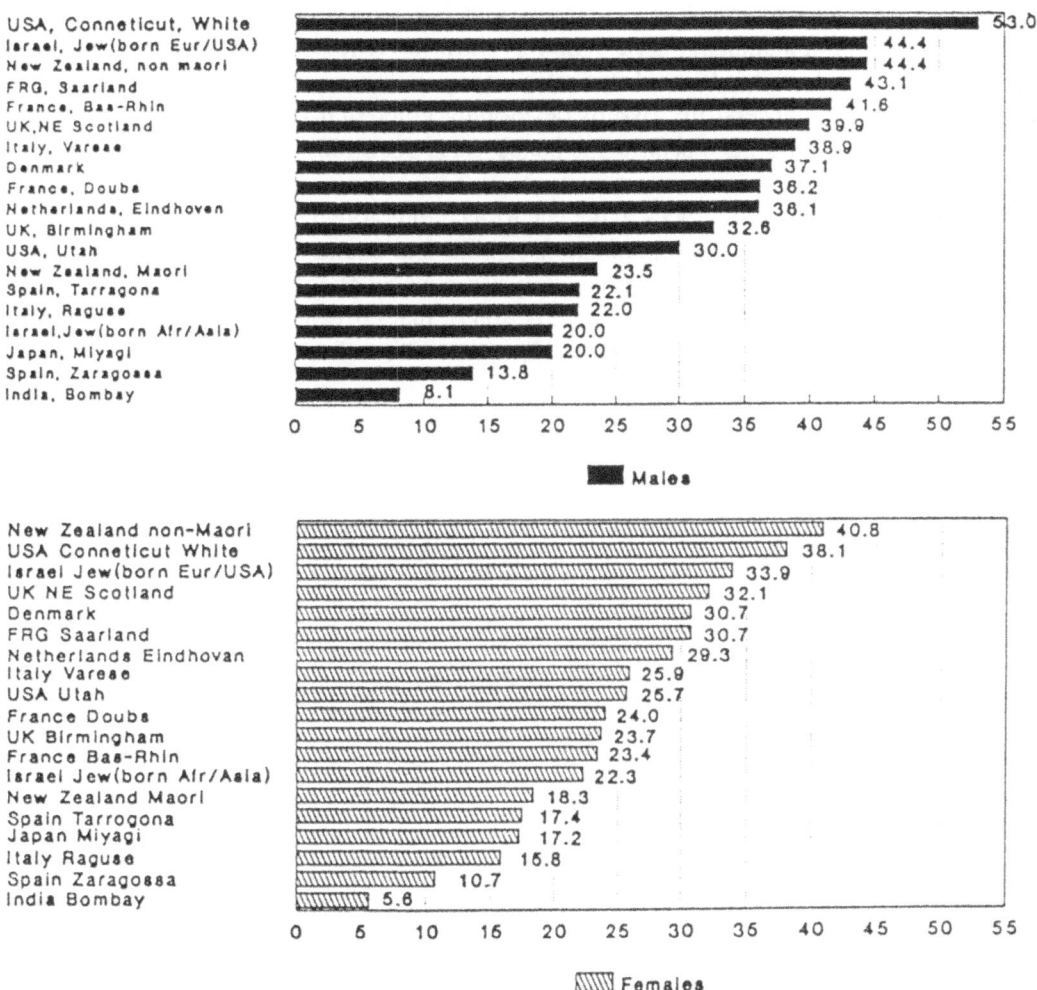

Fig. 2. Average age-standardized (world) incidence rates for cancers of the intestines, chiefly colon and rectum (ICD-9:152-4) per 100,000in selected European Cancer Registry regions and

3

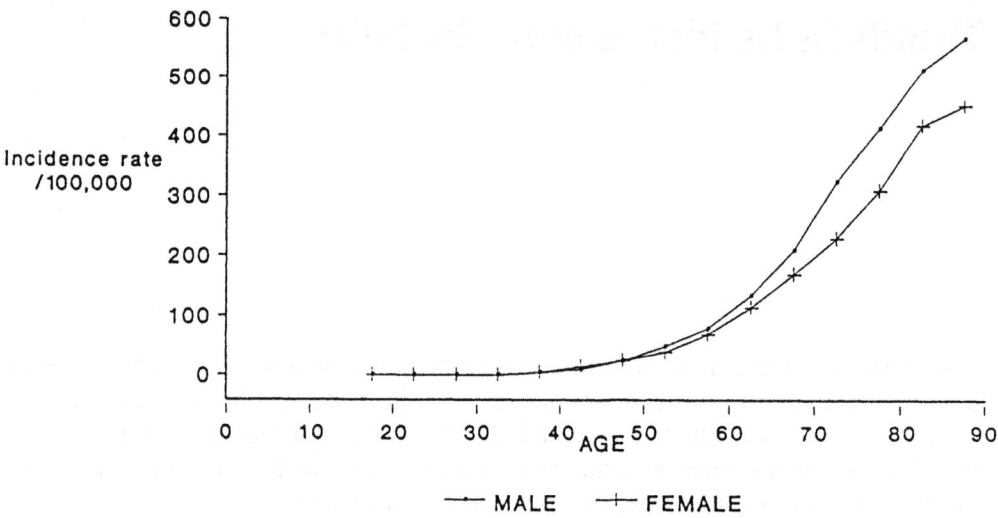

Fig. 3. Age-specific incidence rates of colorectal cancer in Denmark (1978-1982)

by cancer registries. Higher rates than in Europe are found in some North American populations, non-inborn New Zealanders and Israeli Jews of European or American origin. Other populations in these countries show lower rates, mostly in the range of the European registries, while incidence rates from populations in Asia are even lower.

As for most cancers, the risk of developing colorectal cancer increases with age. Figure 3 gives the age-specific incidence rates for colorectal cancer for Denmark (1978-1982).

There are strong differences in the occurrence of colorectal cancer in different ethnic groups or other defined sub-populations within one country. It has also been demonstrated that migrants moving from a low-risk country to a high-risk country increase their risk for colorectal cancer in the direction of that prevailing in the new country and that this change can be seen even in the first generation of migrants.

4

Epidemiology and Aetiology of Colorectal Cancer

Between the cancer registries from EEC countries listed in Figure 2 incidence rates vary up to 3 or 4-fold. Rates are higher in Northern European populations and lower in mediterranian populations. The most obvious difference in the descriptive epidemiology between colonic and rectal cancers is that the male/female ratio is one for colon but in the order of 1.5 to 1.8 for rectal cancer. In addition, the incidence of rectal cancer seems to vary somewhat less internationally than that of colon cancer.

The incidence according to site, sex and age indicates different patterns for the right colon, the left colon and the rectum. In the right colon there appears to be no major difference in incidence by age and sex, for the left colon there is some male predominance, mainly occuring after the age of 65 years, while for the rectum a substantially higher (twofold) incidence is seen in males after the age of 50 years.

Data on Japanese migrants to the United States and European migrants to the United States or Australia demonstrate that the migrant population approach the (high) incidence and mortality figures of the new country of residence. This is taken as strong evidence for the fact that environmental risk factors play an important role in the aetiology of colorectal cancer.

Within one country there can be large differences in the incidence of colorectal cancer between different racial subgroups, for example there is a threefold higher incidence in non-Maori New Zealanders compared to the inborne Maori population. In Hawaii colon cancer rates are higher among Caucasians, Japanese and Chinese compared to Hawaiians and Filipinos (Figure 2).

It has been frequently demonstrated that religious groups which practice lifestyles different from the general population (vegetarian, abstaining from tobacco, alcohol, tea and coffee) experience lower morbidity and mortality from colorectal cancer. Furthermore, colorectal cancer is found somewhat more frequently in higher socio-economic classes. This difference is larger in areas with an overall lower risk. Sedentary occupations have also been associated with a high colorectal cancer risk.

It is obvious that among the environmental risk factors investigated in the aetiology of colorectal cancer dietary habits play a major role. Varying dietary habits between populations, for example, per capita fat consumption, have frequently been used successfully to explain differences in incidence or mortality. However, such an approach would not allow conclusions on a causal relationship, since correlations of aggregate statistics cannot demonstrate "whether those who eat the fat are those who get the cancer". Therefore, studies are necessary relating individual-based dietary information with occurrence or non-occurrence of the disease among these individuals.

Only few studies have been undertaken in which dietary habits have been recorded initially and the disease occurrence observed subsequently. Such prospective cohort studies are considered to provide very valid information. However, they have to be conducted in a large cohort of individuals (several ten thousands) and followed-up for a long period of time.

Studies initiated in the sixties have provided some important clues but did not use a sophisticated methodology of assessing dietary habits. In one cohort study an inverse relationship of saturated fat intake to colon cancer risk was reported, while in another study, also conducted among Japanese population groups, a protective effect of meat consumption as well as consumption of rice against colorectal cancer mortality was reported. Another study did not find any association between dietary fat intake or related nutrients and colon cancer risk. In a study conducted on Seventh Day Adventists some food items (consumption of eggs or coffee) as well as obesity were significantly related to colon cancer mortality.

In a recent prospective cohort study among 90,000 American nurses using validated dietary methodology the risk of developing colorectal cancer was found to be clearly associated with increasing consumption of beef, pork or lamb, as well as dietary fat in general. The latter effect was mainly confined to saturated and monounsaturated fat. In addition, the risk of developing colorectal cancer decreased with increasing consumption of fruits and vegetables or dietary fibre.

In case-control studies newly diagnosed patients with colorectal cancer are interviewed about their past dietary habits and this information compared to that retrieved in a comparable way from non-diseased controls. The validity of retrospectively recalled dietary habits has always been a matter of debate when interpreting the results from such studies. There are some twenty such case-control studies available and most of them indicate an increased risk of colorectal cancer with increasing consumption of meat or fat and decreasing consumption of fruits and vegetables, especially cruciferous vegetables. When dietary fibre has been investigated specifically some studies show a protective effect of fibre consumption whilst others show an increased risk with increasing fibre consumption.

There is strong evidence to support the hypothesis that a diet rich in fat and low in fibre increases the risk for colorectal cancer. This comes from epidemiologic data and there are plausible explanations of a mechanism behind it. These centre around the role of bile acids, the production of which are increased by fat intake but which are more readily bound and excreted by a high fibre content diet. Although the scientific evidence for this is not fully conclusive it has however become practice to include these points in recommendations for a healthy diet. This is not only done for the purpose of preventing colorectal cancer, but these dietary recommendations (low fat, high fibre) are viewed to be of general importance for the maintenance of good health. Specific dietary recommendations for prevention purposes issued by various organisations or bodies advise a reduction of fat intake to about 30% of the daily caloric intake and increase in consumption of fresh fruits and vegetables in order to assure sufficient intake of dietary fibre and vitamins. Avoidance of overweight is a natural consequence. Such recommendations on dietary habits should not be seen in isolation from the advice to abstain from tobacco smoking and moderate the consumption of alcoholic beverages as major lifestyle modifications for the prevention of cancer.

Dietary Risk Factors for Colorectal Cancer	
Factors increasing the risk	Factors decreasing the risk
Consumption of pork & lamb	Consumption of vegetables, especially cruciferous vegetables
Dietary fat (chiefly saturated fatty acids)	Dietary fibre

High Risk Groups

In addition to marked geographical variation in the incidence of colorectal cancer, there are clearly defined groups of people who carry an increased risk of cancer development when compared to the "average" risk in their particular populations. The first of these groups to be recognised was patients with familial adenomatous polyposis (FAP).

Familial Adenomatous Polyposis

The link between multiple polyps in the colo-rectum and carcinoma was first recognised 100 years ago, and while it has long been appreciated that the condition is inherited as an autosomal dominant with high penetrance it is only very recently that the abnormal gene has been located. It is now known that FAP is caused by a single abnormal gene located on the long arm of chromosome 5. While the majority of cases of FAP arise through inheritance of an abnormal gene at this locus, sporadic cases can arise from a new pre-zygotic mutation and the mutated gene will then be passed on to the individual's offspring.

Children of FAP patients have a 50% chance of inheriting the condition, but not all carriers of the

FAP gene will develop the condition. The FAP gene has been identified and it is possible to identify the majority of at risk individuals who can be regularly screened for the development of polyposis. Furthermore, 75-80% of FAP gene carriers exhibit congenital hypertrophy of retinal pigment epithelial (CHRPE) which can be detected on ophthalmological examination.

Adenomas usually develop during the first two or three decades of life and 92% of those individuals destined to develop FAP will manifest the disease by the age of 30 years. Their development should be sought by yearly fibreoptic sigmoidoscopy commencing at the age of 15 years. If negative findings on endoscopy are combined with a favourable result from an investigation of linked gene markers, and an absence of CHRPE, then the residual risk of development of the disease can become very low, for example 1 in 1000 at age 30 years.

Individuals who do develop FAP will, if not treated, inevitably progress to colorectal carcinoma. In order to prevent this development prophylactic surgery must be undertaken. In the past the majority of cases have been treated by total colectomy with ileo-rectal anastomosis followed by regular examination of the retained rectum. However, this operation (despite surveillance) carries an appreciable risk of rectal cancer, and there is an increasing trend towards restorative proctocolectomy with an ileo-anal pouch anastomosis. This preserves anatomical continuity while totally eliminating the at risk large bowel mucosa.

For many years FAP was considered to be a disease solely affecting the large intestine. When extra-intestinal lesions were encountered in association with FAP they were categorised into a multiplicity of separate syndromes, the best known being Gardner's syndrome where the patients have desmoids, epidermoid cysts and osteomas in addition to FAP. It is now believed that all these syndromes represent different modes of expression of the FAP gene in which multiple adenomatous polyps are the common denominator.

A recently recognised aspect of FAP is the high incidence and potential danger of upper gastrointestinal lesions and desmoid tumours. Polyps in the stomach are a frequent finding, but these are usually non-neoplastic and can be ignored. Much more serious is the development of duodenal adenomas which exhibit the same malignant potential as colorectal adenomas but are more difficult to eradicate.

Duodenal cancer, particularly peri-ampullary cancer, is an importrant cause of death in FAP patients.

Screening of Relatives in Fap Families
Yearly fibreoptic sigmoidoscopy after age 15 years Genetic markers CHRPE sought by ophthalmological examination

Other Polyposis Syndromes

Two other syndromes in which there is an increased risk of malignancy are *Peutz-Jeghers polyposis* and *multiple juvenile polyposis*. Peutz-Jeghers polyps are usually classified as congenital malformations (hamartomas) and formerly have not been considered to carry a risk of malignant change. Certainly, such polyps rarely if ever show cytological atypia. Nevertheless, recent studies appear to show an increased incidence of gastrointestinal cancer in this condition, albeit mainly in the stomach and small intestine. The increased risk, however, is small and a conservative approach to surgical management is advocated. Multiple juvenile polyps are much less commonly found than sporadic or isolated juvenile polyps which can be considered totally benign. Examination of polyps from multiple polyposis cases however reveals a small proportion showing malignant change. Thus this condition, although a rarity, is thought to carry an increased risk of colorectal cancer, but clear guidelines for its management have not yet emerged.

Hereditary Non-Polyposis Colorectal Cancer (HNPCC)

Separate from individuals with multiple polyposis, there are well recognised familial clusters of colorectal cancer as part of the so-called "family cancer syndrome". These fall into two main categories. Firstly, where large bowel cancer is found within families who also exhibit a high incidence of other adenocarcinomas, for example, breast, endometrium and stomach. Secondly, there are other families who exhibit clustering of colorectal cancer alone. In both instances, the cancers are found at a younger age (around 40 years), they are more often multiple, and there is a preponderance of right sided tumours. It is probable that these two patterns result from an identical genetic abnormality transmitted as an autosomal dominant but modified by different environmental factors. It seems likely that patients inherit a susceptibility to adenomas and that they exhibit the same adenoma-carcinoma sequence as FAP patients. In accordance with this hypothesis, adenomas in HNPCC families are of larger size, and show a greater villous pattern and more cytological abnormalities (dysplasia) than sporadic adenomas.

Relatives with Colorectal Cancer

Although FAP and HNPCC only account for about 5% of all colorectal cancers, a more important role for hereditary factors is suggested by the finding that 20-25% of patients with large bowel cancer have at least one first degree relative who is similarly affected even though no well-defined inheritance pattern can be determined. Furthermore, there is a significantly increased frequency of adenomas in relatives compared to spouse-controls, and these adenomas are more numerous and larger than controls. One large study has calculated the risk of colorectal cancer among relatives of patients with adenocarcinoma to be 2.4 times greater than in normal individuals, but the risk is considerably increased if an individual has more than one first degree relative with colorectal cancer, particularly if the cancer occurred before the age of 45y (8-25% lifetime risk).

Previous Adenoma or Carcinoma

Patients who have had a previous adenoma or a previous cancer are at increased risk of developing a subsequent neoplasm. Between 20 and 40% of patients who have an adenoma removed will develop subsequent adenomas within 10 years of the index polypectomy, the risk being highest for patients having multiple rather than single adenomas at first presentation. Approximately 5% of patients who have undergone a curative resection for colorectal carcinoma will develop a further large bowel cancer within 10 years of operation. The increased risk is however, life-long and this, together with the propensity for subsequent (metachronous) cancers to arise in the right colon underlines the need for assessment of the entire colon in the follow-up of colorectal cancer patients.

Long-standing Ulcerative Colitis

Ulcerative colitis (UC) has long been recognised as a condition pre-disposing to the development of colorectal cancer. Most early studies tended to overestimate the degree of risk, calculating cumulative cancer rates ranging from 16% to 43%, depending on the duration of disease. It is now clear that the risk is lower than this, and an overall figure of 10% at 20 years from onset is more realistic. Nevertheless, there is a substantial increased risk with total colitis versus distal colitis/proctitis, and this risk is sufficient to warrant surveillance of patients with extensive and long-standing UC even if their symtpoms are minimal. Such surveillance, colonoscopy and biopsy, should be instituted 8-10 years after onset.

Other Pre-disposing Conditions

While it is firmly established that uretero-colic anastomoses (performed usually for bladder cancer) pre-disposes to colonic cancer there is speculation that other surgical procedures such as gastric surgery and cholecystectomy are associated with an increased risk of the subsequent development of colorectal cancer. The excess risk following these operations is small, and some authorities would dispute their role.

High risk groups
Familial adenomatous polyposis – Hereditary non-polyposis colorectal cancer – Close relatives with colorectal cancer – Previous adenoma or colorectal cancer – Long-standing extensive ulcerative colitis Other polyposis syndromes: – Peutz-Jeghers polyposis – Multiple juvenile polyposis

Role of Inheritance and Environment

On the basis of recent family pedigree studies it can be proposed that the majority of colorectal neoplasms arise in individuals with an inherited susceptibility to adenomas. It is clear, however, that environmental factors play a central role in the development of adenomas in susceptible individuals and in their progression to carcinoma. Thus the interplay of hereditary and environment can occur at several levels.

1) In individuals who inherit the FAP gene, the development of adenomas is solely under genetic control but the subsequent progression to carcinoma (which takes 10-15 years) is probably influenced by environmental factors which lead to further mutational events.

2) In many individuals (including HNPCC families) there is an inherited susceptibility to adenoma formation, but neoplasia only develops when triggering environmental factors result in a genetic mutation, probably at the chromosome 5 locus. Further mutations, frequently affecting *oncogenes* which control cell growth and differentiation, and partial chromosome deletions in which tumour suppressor genes are lost, lead to the formation of a sub-clone of malignant cells in the adenoma and an invasive carcinoma develops.

3) In unusual circumstances an increased carcinogenic load in the gut lumen could cause mutations and allele deletions which initiate the adenoma-carcinoma sequence in non-susceptible (normal) gut mucosa. This could be facilitated by the promotional effects of increased cell turnover as found for example in inflammatory bowel disease, but could also result from dietary factors. In such individuals hereditary factors may not be operative.

Adenomas

The majority of colorectal carcinomas arise from pre-existing adenomas. Adenomas are very common and only a small proportion undergo malignant change; many are detected either clinically or by screening and are removed prior to the development

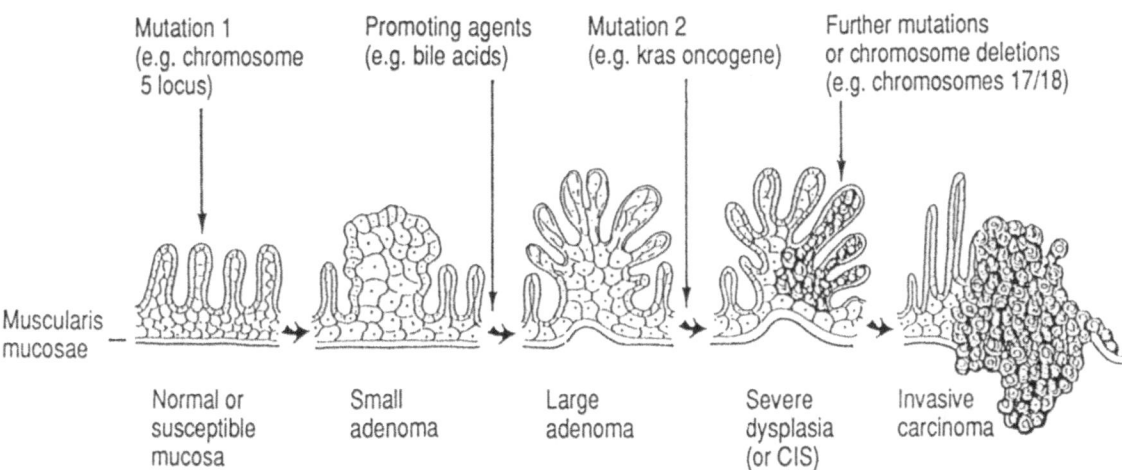

Fig. 4. Multistep theory of carcinogenesis

of carcinoma, whilst many which remain undetected persist as adenomas up to death. These observations are consistent with different factors being responsible for adenoma formation and carcinomatous change, and are in keeping with the multistep theory of carcinogenesis (Figure 4).

An adenoma is a neoplastic proliferation of epithelial cells, derived from a single precursor cell, the cells exhibit varying degrees of cytological abnormality (dysplasia) and form, along with connective tissue stroma, a protuberant lesion showing two main histological growth patterns, *tubular* - where crypt profiles predominate, or *villous* - where the epithelium is thrown into elongated, finger-like processes. At the gross level, adenomas can be broad based or *sessile* or on a stalk of uninvolved mucosa - *pedunculated*. Small tubular adenomas are frequently pedunculated, whereas large adenomas (particularly villous adenomas) are generally sessile.

Factors Associated with Malignant Change

In general as adenomas increase in size they show an increasing incidence of malignant change. Increasing size is associated with a more villous pattern and increasing dysplasia, and the latter feature is closely related to malignancy.

The cytological and architectural abnormalities comprising dysplasia are usually classified into mild, moderate and severe. In colorectal adenomas the term *severe dysplasia* is synonymous with *carcinoma-in-situ* (CIS) and is applied when the epithelial cells have a "malignant" morphology but show no invasion through the basement membrane. When invasion into the connective tissue of the mucosa (lamina propria) is seen, this could be termed *intramucosal carcinoma*. In practice, this term is generally avoided by European histopathologists as carcinoma limited to the colorectal mucosa is not biologically "malignant", that is, it will not metastasise and kill the patient. In view of this, such lesions are usually included within the *severe dysplasia* or *carcinoma-in-situ* category. The benign behaviour of this superficial lamina propria invasion relates to the lymphatic drainage of the colorectal mucosa which only commences in a plexus in the deep mucosa close to the muscularis mucosae. Thus, carcinoma

cells have to reach and penetrate the muscularis mucosae before the lesion can be considered truly malignant. Histological reporting of these early changes is subject to differing terminologies, but it is generally acknowledged that invasion through the muscularis mucosae (*submucosal* or *invasive carcinoma*) is the stage at which a metastatic risk develops. Between 2% and 8% of all colorectal polyps removed endoscopically will exhibit such invasive carcinoma, but its prevalence is very dependent upon size. Adenomas less than 10 mm in diameter exhibit a very low frequency of invasive carcinoma (less than 0.5%) whereas about 5% of adenomas measuring between 11 and 20 mm and 10% of those greater than 20 mm diameter show malignant change.

Metastatic potential has a great bearing on the management of polyps. After polypectomy, adenomas showing severe dysplasia or carcinoma-in-situ can be considered biologically non-aggressive and no further treatment is required. Even with invasion of the submucosa, polypectomy is generally curative. Adverse factors which point to a high-risk of cancer recurrence relate to inadequate removal or an increased risk of metastasis; these are involvement of the polyp base by carcinoma cells (or widespread invasion close to the cut margin), lymphatic permeation and poor differentiation. Involvement of the base is much more likely with sessile rather than pedunculated polyps. Patients whose adenomas exhibit these adverse factors should undergo surgical resection of the segment containing the polyp base together with lymph node dissection.

Risk of Metastases in Malignant Polyps	
Stage of malignant change	Risk of metastasis
Severe dysplasia Carcinoma-in-situ	None
Invasice carcinoma (that is invasion into the submucosa)	About 10% have regional lymph node involvement

Symptoms

Colorectal cancer usually presents with symptoms late in its natural history. Symptoms and signs are not specific, but are usually the consequence of narrowing of the bowel luman producing sub-acute obstruction or by the loss of blood or mucus from the tumour surface resulting in a change in bowel habit. Less frequently the patient presents with systemic symptoms of tiredness and malaise due to anaemia or due to the presence of distant metastases. The relevance of clinical symptoms depends upon the association of two or more of them and the timing of their onset. For example, overt rectal bleeding lasting several years and characterized by small amounts of fresh blood at the end of evacuation is more suggestive of haemorrhoids than cancer, but even then it requires thorough investigation. A long lasting bowel irregularity, characterized by alternating constipation with diarrhoea is suggestive of irritable bowel syndrome (IBS), but arising for the first time in elderly patients is more suggestive of a colonic neoplasm.

The type of symptoms and their frequency varies with the anatomical location of the tumour within the large bowel.

Right Colon

In the right colon as the bowel lumen is large and the stools are liquid, obstructive symptoms are unusual. In this situation tumours can grow to a large size without producing symptoms and commonly present as a mass in the abdomen. Likewise, chronic iron deficiency anaemia may result from the blood loss from the tumour surface without obvious blood being seen in the faeces. A patient may also present with weight loss and fever. Occasionally obstructive symptoms are produced by the tumour involving the ileal caecal valve or the opening of the appendix.

Left Colon

In the left colon where the bowel lumen is small and the stools more solid, obstructive symptoms are commonly found, the common symptom being a change of bowel habit with alternating diarrhoea and constipation. This may be assoicated with left-sided lower abdominal colicky pain or discomfort. Rectal bleeding with or without mucus in the stool is also frequent.

Rectum

Rectal bleeding and a change in the type of stool passed is a common symptom, the blood is characteristically mixed in the stool, whereas the blood from haemorrhoidal bleeding is often separate from the stool and sometimes splashed on the sides of the toilet bowl. However, rectal bleeding should only be attributed to haemorrhoids after careful investigation has excluded neoplastic lesions in the rectum.

Other symptoms include tenesmus, a sense of incomplete evacuation and a change in the shape of the stool. Tumours involving the anal canal also present with anal discomfort.

Many benign colonic diseases such as diverticular disease, irritable bowel syndrome and inflammatory bowel disease are associated with symptoms very similar to that of colorectal cancer, exclusion of cancer in these patients is therefore necessary.

Investigations

Physical Examination and Rectal Examination

The patient should be examined for signs of anaemia, abdominal masses, irregular enlargement of the liver. Approximately 70% of rectal cancers are within reach of the examining finger. However, small early rectal neoplasms, particularly those that are polypoidal may be difficult to feel and negative rectal examinations should not deter further investigations being carried out.

Endoscopy

Endoscopy by fibreoptic instruments is today the procedure of choice for the examination of the large bowel. It allows direct visualization of the bowel, biopsy of suspicious lesions and the removal of polyps by snare polypectomy.

Rigid sigmoidoscopy can only be relied upon only to examine the rectum to the level of 15 cm. It is often impossible to pass the instrument beyond this distance because of angulation of the rectosigmoid junction. Investigation is simple to perform without the necessity of bowel preparation. The majority of rectal cancers can be diagnosed. The examination is useful in excluding other causes of bleeding such as proctitis. A negative rectoscopy in the presence of symptoms indicates the need for further investigation.

Flexible sigmoidoscopy allows direct inspection of the distal large bowel, the site of occurrence of most colorectal cancers. The 60 cm instrument is able to detect 50 - 60% of colorectal cancers and a similar proportion of large adenomas. Flexible sigmoidoscopy has better subject acceptance compared with rigid sigmoidoscopy but some simple method of bowel preparation is usually required.

Colonoscopy performed by a trained endoscopist provides optimum examination in symptomatic patients and in asymptomatic individuals with a positive faecal occult blood test or other high risk condition. A further advantage of colonoscopy is that the examination may be therapeutic as adenomatous polyps can be removed by polypectomy at the time of the examination and additional synchronous lesions may be detected. Small polypoidal lesions may be missed by colonoscopy even in skilled hands. Complications such as perforation are usually associated with therapeutic manipulation such as polypectomy, in diagnostic examinations the risk is very low.

Radiology

Air contrast studies of the large bowel were introduced to overcome the limitations of conventional barium enema. The double contrast barium enema is the only reliable radiological diagnostic investigation for neoplastic disease of the large bowel. Sensitivity for detecting small polypoidal lesions on double contrast barium enema is less than that of colonoscopy, particularly in the sigmoid colon in the presence of diverticular disease. Double contrast barium enema is well tolerated and safe. In the absence of skilled colonoscopic expertise, double contrast barium enema and flexible sigmoidoscopy are an alternative method of examinating the whole colon.

Laboratory Faecal Occult Blood Testing

Faecal occult blood testing has a limited role in the investigation of symptomatic individuals. A positive Haemoccult test identifies individuals with a greater likelihood of harbouring a colorectal neoplasm. Colonoscopy is the most appropriate method of investigation of patients known to have a positive occult blood test.

Screening for Colorectal Cancer

Screening represents an alternative possibility of influencing the mortality of colorectal cancer in a population. It may reduce mortality in two ways. Firstly by the detection of tumours early in their natural history before they have produced symptoms and when the tumour is amenable to surgical treatment and secondly, by the detection and removal of premalignant adenomas with a resulting decrease in the future incidence of colorectal cancer.

Colorectal cancer fulfills many of the requirements that are necessary before screening can be expected to improve the outcome of the disease. It is a common tumour, the treatment of tumours at a less advanced pathological stage is more successful, and it is possible to identify persons at an increased risk of development of the disease (See page 4-7). In population screening the most important risk determinant is the age of the patient, the incidence of colorectal cancer rising sharply after the age of 45 and continuing to increase approximately two-fold in each subsequent decade.

Screening Methods

The performance of a screening test is described in terms of sensitivity and specificity. The sensitivity of a test is the proportion of persons with the disease in whom the test is positive. Specificity of the test is the proportion of unaffected people in the population in whom the test is negative. The predictive value of a positive test is the proportion of individuals tested as positive who actually have the disease.

Faecal Occult Blood Tests

The stool of normal persons contains small amounts of blood. An increased blood loss has been shown to occur in patients with colorectal neoplasia. There is however, considerable variation from day to day making it necessary to test individuals for several days. In patients with small adenomas the stool/haemoglobin concentration is usually within normal limits but in patients with large adenomas, a blood loss similar to that of cancer is often found.

The Hemoccult impregnated guaiac slide test for blood in the stool was introduced 20 years ago as a screen for colorectal cancer. It is based on the oxidation of a naturally occurring phenolic chromogen of guaiaconic acid to quinone structure which has a blue colour. Hydrogen peroxide is used as the oxidizing agent and the reaction is catalysed by peroxidases and by haematin. The test is undertaken on two samples of stool for three consecutive days. The test is not specific and vegetable peroxidase in the stool can result in a positive test. Elimination of meat and high peroxidase containing vegetables from the diet will improve the specificity. More specific tests for blood have been introduced in recent years. The Hemoquant test measures the total blood loss from the gastrointestinal tract and a meat free diet is therefore essential. Immunological tests for human blood are selective for lower gut bleeding as the protein part of haemoglobin loses its antigenicity as it is digested during passage through the small bowel. A number of such tests have been evaluated and although they have a greater sensitivity for neoplasia, the cost is greater and more technical expertise is required to perform them, their specificity in population screening has yet to be fully evaluated.

Investigation of Persons with a Positive Faecal Occult Blood Test

Persons found to have a positive test should be investigated by colonoscopy or if the expertise and facilities are not available, by flexible sigmoidoscopy and double contrast barium enema.

Evaluation of Screening Programmes

In the Federal Republic of Germany, screening for colorectal cancer was introduced in 1977 using Hemoccult and rectal digital examination. The acceptance of this screening test has been disappointingly low, but there is evidence that cancers detected are at an earlier stage of their natural history. Four randomised trials of colorectal screening are being undertaken in Europe.

The data from these trials show that tumours detected by screening are at a less advanced pathological stage than when compared with cancers in symptomatic patients. In the Nottingham and Funen trial (Table 2), 52% of screen detected cancers are localised to the bowel (Dukes' Stage A) whereas in the unscreened control group only 10-12% of cancers are at this favourable stage. Only 4% of screen detected patients are found to have liver secondaries at the time of surgery compared with 23% of symptomatic patients. It should also be noted that 16-18% of invasive cancers detected by screening can be removed by endoscopic polypectomy compared with only 0-1.6% of symptomatic cancers. It is likely that reliable mortality data from the European control trials of faecal occult blood testing will not be available until 1994/95.

Table 2. Comparison of cancers detected in Nottingham and Funen control trials

	Nottingham trial Screen detected cancer (n = 122)	Control Group cancer (n = 261)
% Stage A	51.0%	12.0%
% Liver metastases	5.7%	21.8%
% Colonoscopic polypectomy	18.5%	1.6%

	Funen trial (n = 49)	(n = 95)
% Stage A	51.0%	9.0%
% Liver metastase	3.5%	23.5%
% Colonoscopic polypectomy	16.0%	0.0%

Endoscopic Screening

Flexible sigmoidoscopy should replace rigid sigmoidoscopy for colorectal cancer screening because of the greater yield of neoplasia and better patient acceptance. Screening by colonoscopy should be limited to high risk patients.

Screening Recommendations

Until reliable mortality data is available from the European control trials, population screening should only be undertaken in the context of a controlled trial or as part of an evaluation of a new screening

Table 1. European controlled trials of Hemoccult in screening for colorectal cancer

	Cohort Size	Positivity rate(%)	Predictive value (%) (adenomas & cancer)
Goteborg, Sweden	27,000	1.9	22
Nottingham, England	150,000	2.1	53
Odense, Denmark	62,000	1.0	58
Burgundy, France	47,150	2.1	44

test. Average risk individuals who request screening should be screened by one or two yearly Haemoccult testing and 3-5 yearly fibreoptic sigmoidoscopy.

Average risk

1 - 2 yearly Hemoccult and 3 - 5 yearly flexible sigmoidoscopy

High risk

More than two first degree relatives)
Hereditary non-polyposis syndrome)Colonoscopy
Long standing extensive ulcerative

Treatment

Adenomatous Polyps

Endoscopic Polypectomy

Polyps greater than 1 cm in size are usually adenomas, whereas polyps less than 5 mm are usually hyperplastic and not neoplastic in most cases. Adenomas are considered to be precancerous. However, only 5-10% of the adenomas develop into cancer and the process may take several years. Cancer very seldom develops without a preceding adenoma. The risk of a cancer being present within an adenoma increases with the size of the adenoma.

Accordingly, all polyps should be removed and this may be achieved in most cases by endoscopic polypectomy. Large sessile adenomas need surgical removal. Other reasons for removing polyps are symptoms such as bleeding, changed bowel habits and protrusion through the anus.

When an adenoma is detected, there is a 30% risk of another being present in the colon; this justifies a complete colonoscopy to secure a clean colon. Small polyps left behind may grow and follow-up endoscopy is recommended.

Most adenomas do not give any symptoms and are detected by examinations for other suspected diseases. Large polyps over 2 cm in diameter may cause occult bleeding which may be chemically detected in 70% of the cases, but they may also produce the same symptoms as cancer.

Polypectomy may be performed by electrocautery snaring of the polyp-stalk, piecemeal electrocautery snaring of sessile polyps above 1cm in diameter and hot biopsy of small sessile polyps below 5 mm in diameter. Hot biopsy causes destruction of the polyp, but also results in a biopsy, which is considered satisfactory in these small polyps which very rarely contain cancer and probably have a low potency for later malignancy. Ordinary biopsy should not be used. It is very often not representative for the whole polyp and makes later complete polypectomy more difficult. Also the risk of bleeding is higher than after electrocautery.

There is a small risk of complications from endoscopic polypectomy. Intestinal perforation and bleeding from the polyp site may occur. Symptoms of an acute abdomen or visible bleeding should always result in immediate referral to hospital. However, complications from endoscopic polypectomy are much less common than those following laparotomy with polypectomy through a colotomy.

Adenomas containing cancer may also be treated by hot snare polypectomy, provided that the pathologist can verify that the carcinoma has been removed completely and that the resection line is free of carcinoma. If the polyp is less than 2-3 cm in diameter, very few of these patients will have regional lymph node metastases. However, sessile adenomas with carcinoma should generally be treated by surgery because it is not possible to be sure that the carcinoma has been completely removed by applying the piecemeal technique.

Adenomas removed by endoscopic procedures found to have carcinoma at or close to resection margin, vascular or lymphatic invasion, or poor differentiation should be treated further by surgical resection. Endoscopic polypectomy only carries a small risk of complications and is safer than surgical removal.

Follow-up After Adenoma Removal

This follow-up aims at reducing the risk of developing cancer by detecting overlooked and incompletely removed adenomas during the first 3 months, and later the development of new adenomas.

Clean Colon Secured by Total Colonoscopy:

50% Risk of New Adenomas Within 10 Years

Colonoscopy is the optimal way of securing a clean colon, but colonoscopy may not always be available, making less optimal examinations such as flexible sigmoidoscopy plus double contrast barium enema (DCBE), or even rigid proctoscopy plus DCBE acceptable. The traditional barium enema should not be used, because of a very low accuracy for detecting early neoplasia. It may not always be possible to reach the caecum by colonoscopy because of diverticular disease or intraperitoneal adhesions. The examination must then be supplemented by DCBE. Early follow-up is necessary after piece-meal removal of large sessile adenomas, because the pathologist can seldom guarantee complete removal, following extensive fulguration of the base of the polyp and cancer may be missed. Colonoscopy should also be repeated within 3 months in patients with multiple polyps as the risk of overlooking adenomas is high and also the endoscopist may have left adenomas behind on purpose because of the long period of time used for the initial removal of many polyps.

Large controlled trials to evaluate benefit from long term follow-up are underway in the USA and Denmark. The intervals between examinations should probably be 3 to 4 years, but subgroups such as those with villous adenomas and multiple adenomas may need shorter intervals because of higher risk of new adenomas. Tests for occult bleeding like the Hemoccult-II test may be performed every second year to reduce the risk of overlooking fast growing cancers.

Retrospective studies suggest that repeated rectoscopies in patients with rectal adenomas will decrease the incidence of rectal cancer but this remains to be confirmed in prospective trials for colonic as well as rectal adenomas.

At the present time it seems justified to recommend colorectal examination by colonoscopy every 3 to 4 years in patients being fit for any follow-up, ie excluding patients with severe complicating disease, or disease which makes follow-up inconvenient to the patient. It should be remembered that even diagnostic colonoscopy and DCBE carry small risks of intestinal perforation.

Follow-up After Adenoma Removal

Within 3 months to secure that adenoma and even carcinoma is not left behind

Later, to detect and remove new adenomas

Surgical Treatment

Surgery remains the cornerstone of treatment for colorectal cancer. In the last 50 years, the operability rate has gradually increased in most colorectal units to 95%. With improvements in anaesthesia, antibiotics, fluid and electrolyte balance, elective surgery for the disease is relatively safe. Unfortunately, not all patients with the disease reach the surgeon; a proportion die from complications before surgical treatment can be undertaken. Although the operability rate has steadily improved, the 5-year survival rate has remained static at approximately 50% of all patients undergoing an apparent curative resection. The challenge in the future will be to improve on this figure.

Pre-operative Investigations and Preparation

Once the diagnosis has been made, it is important to assess the patient carefully; first with regard to the extent of spread of the carcinoma and second, to determine the fitness of the patient for surgery.

Each patient should have the liver scanned, preferably by CT, but if this is not available, by ultrasound; a chest X-ray should also be performed. If metastases are present, then surgery will be palliative rather than curative. Ideally, a colonoscopy or barium enema should be carried out before an operation is performed. Approximately 3% of patients with a colorectal cancer have a second or third synchronous carcinoma at the time of presentation, and 20% have adenomatous polyps. Unfortunately some growths are constricting in nature, and it is not possible either on radiology or endoscopy to obtain a satisfactory view of the colon proximal to them. In these circumstances the appropriate investigations should be performed, either peroperatively or within 6 months of the operation. The serum CEA concentration is useful in assessing the likelihood of metastases. For rectal carcinoma, it is useful to assess the extent of local spread by pelvic CT or endoluminal ultrasound. Infiltration of local structures is not a contra-indication for surgery, but in some centres is an indication for pre-operative radiotherapy. The latter has the ability to reduce the size of a carcinoma, and convert it from an inoperable to an operable lesion. An intravenous urography may be required to assess renal function, particularly for patients with a left-sided tumour which might infiltrate the left ureter. Although this investigation is no longer recommended as routine, it is helpful to know that the kidney on the opposite side is functioning should it be necessary to remove the one on the affected side.

PreOperative Investigations
Chest X-ray
Liver CT or US
Barium enema or colonoscopy
Serum CEA
Endoluminal US or Pelvic CT for rectal cancer (if available)

All tumours should, if possible, be biopsied before surgery to confirm the diagnosis. The biopsies can be graded according to the degree of histological differentiation. In the past, the type of operation to be performed for a rectal carcinoma was influenced by the degree of differentiation of the tumour. Thus, poorly differentiated rectal cancers were treated by an abdomino-perineal excision of the rectum (APER). However, it has now been shown that a pre-operative biopsy is inaccurate in predicting the histological grade of the tumour, and such a policy has been abandoned.

Principles of Surgical Resection

Provided the patient is deemed fit enough to undergo a laparotomy, a resection of the affected portion of the large bowel should be carried out. The patient needs bowel preparation before operation to reduce the risks of faecal contamination of the peritoneal cavity and anastomotic breakdown. This is usually carried out by a mixture of laxatives, enemas and rectal washouts. Antibiotic prophylaxis and subcutaneous heparin administration should be used to reduce the risk of post-operative sepsis and deep venous thrombosis respectively.

The extent of colorectal resection will depend on the site of the tumour. The principle is to remove the segment of bowel containing the tumour and its associated lymphatic drainage; since the lymphatic drainage follows the blood supply the extent of resection depends on the viability of the remaining bowel. Over the years, the various operations for colon cancer have been standardised and are illustrated in Figure 5-8. It is usual to establish gastroin-

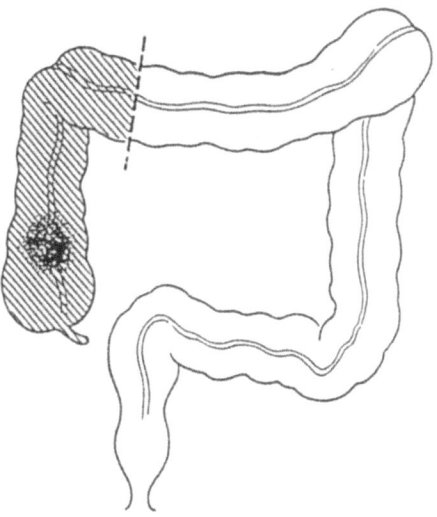

Fig. 5. Right hemicolectomy

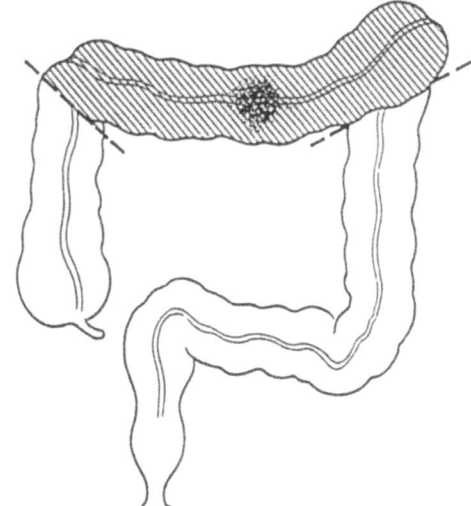

Fig. 6. Transverse colectomy

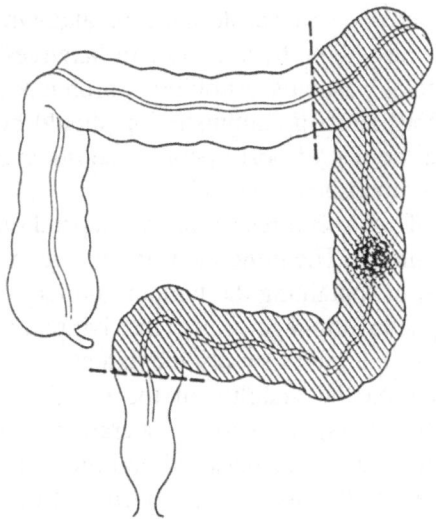

Fig. 7. Left hemicolectomy

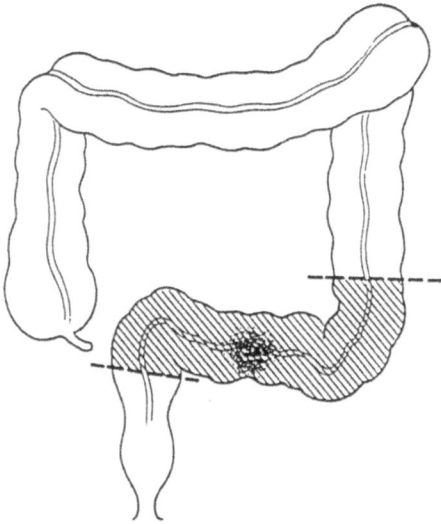

Fig. 8. Sigmoid colectomy

testinal continuity by ileo-colic, colo-colic or colo-rectal anastomosis unless there has been some septic complication, and in such cases it is usual to exteriorise one or both ends of bowel and anastomose at a later date. Excision of the tumour must be aggressive if at all possible, even if this means resecting part or all of involved visci. Often the tumour adheres to other organs like the small intestine, and an en bloc resection is required. In approximately 25% of patients who appear to have malignant infiltration into other organs, the pathological report shows the tumour to be attached to them by an inflammatory response. In such cases the prognosis is as good as tumours which are mobile and non-invasive.

Rectal Carcinoma

The surgical treatment of rectal cancer has undergone a revolution in the last decade, with the emphasis on anal sphincter preservation. A rectal carcinoma spreads upwards, downwards and laterally, and it was for this reason that Miles in 1908 developed the operation of abdomino-perineal excision (Figure 9). In this operation, which nowadays is synchonously performed by two surgeons, the rectum, the sigmoid colon, the mesorectum, the anal sphincter and the ischiorectal fat are removed, the perineum is closed and a permanent left iliac fossa is constructed (Figure 10). For many years, this operation was performed for all rectal cancers no matter where they were sited within the rectum. Then in the 1940's, some surgeons began to treat patients with tumours of the upper third of the rectum by anterior resection. In this operation the tumour and upper third of rectum were excised and the descending colon was anastomosed to the middle third of the rectum (Figure 11). Gradually surgeons became bolder and extended the operation to treat suitable patients with tumours of the middle third of the rectum. However, there was a limit to how far down in the pelvis an anstomosis could be constructed by hand. In addition, there were theorectical reasons why it was considered that anterior resection should not be pushed to the limit of the surgeon's expertise. It was thought that at least 6-8 cm of anorectum needed to be retained if normal anorectal function was to be adequate, and it was also believed that at least 5 cm of normal distal rectum needed to be removed with the specimen to prevent local recurrence from microscopic intramural distal spread.

In the last decade, this whole philosophy has changed. Techniques have been developed to achieve an anstomosis at a much lower level in the pelvis than was ever previously envisaged. Most notable amongst these techniques has been the use of the circular stapling gun, which permits a secure stapled anastomosis to be constructed between the colon and anorectal stump in two layers, without direct visualisation by the surgeon (Figure 12). Pari passu with the development has been the realisation that provided certain precautions are taken, continence and relatively normal function can be achieved, despite the reduction in length of the anorectal stump to a few centimetres. Similarly patho-

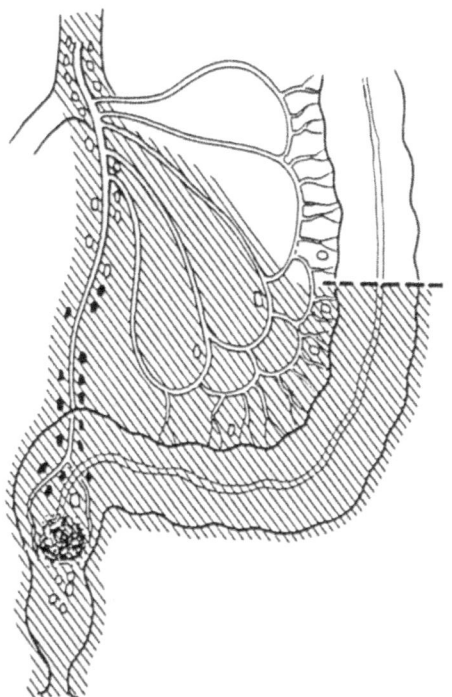

Fig. 9. Abdomino-perineal resection

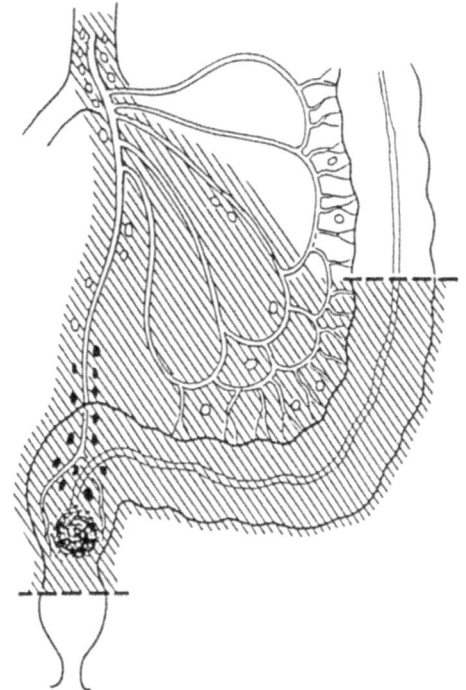

Fig. 11. Anterior restorative resection

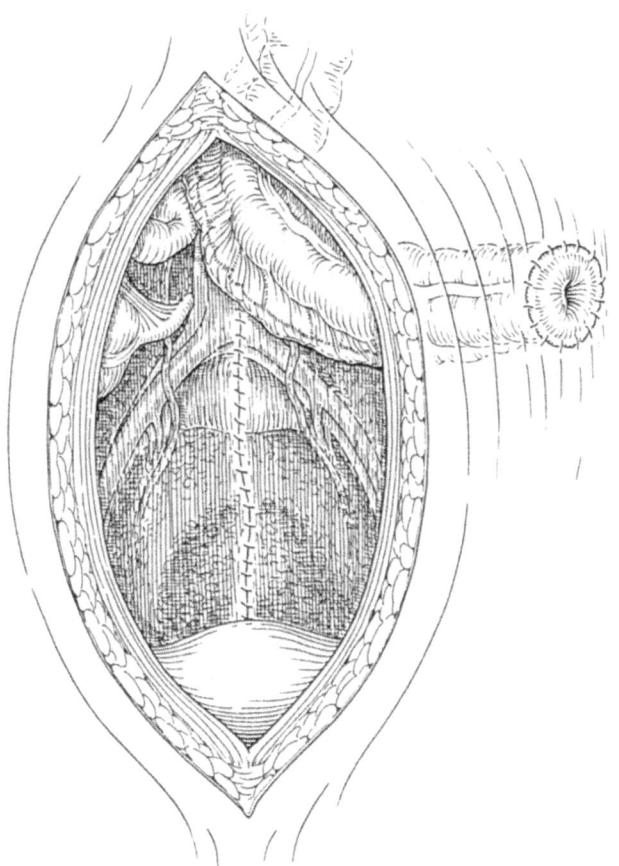

Fig. 10. Formation of colostomy after abdomino-perineal resection

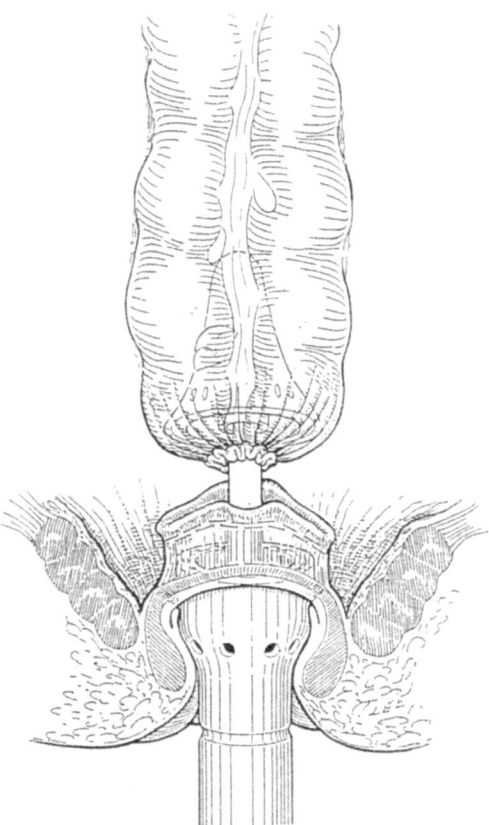

Fig. 12. Stapled anastomosis after anterior resection

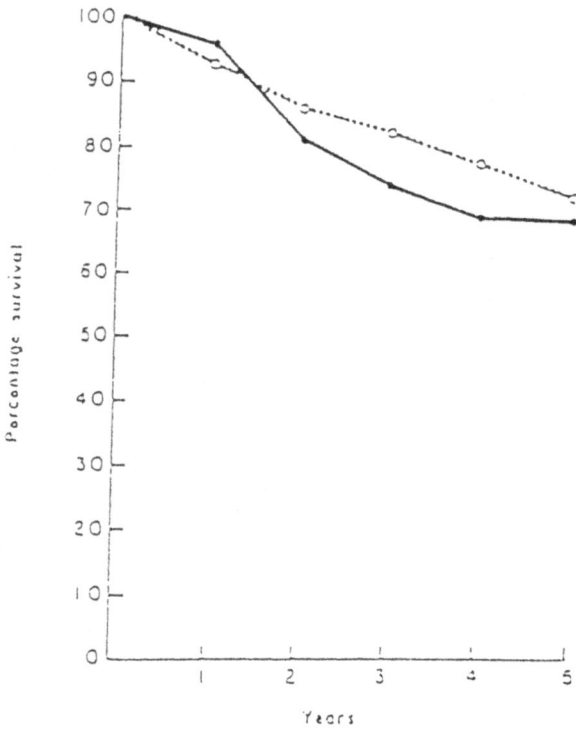

Fig. 13. Corrected 5 year survival curves for restorative anterior resection o---o and for abdominoperineal excision **o---o** (Reproduced from The British Journal of Surgery 72:597 by permission of Butterworth & Co)

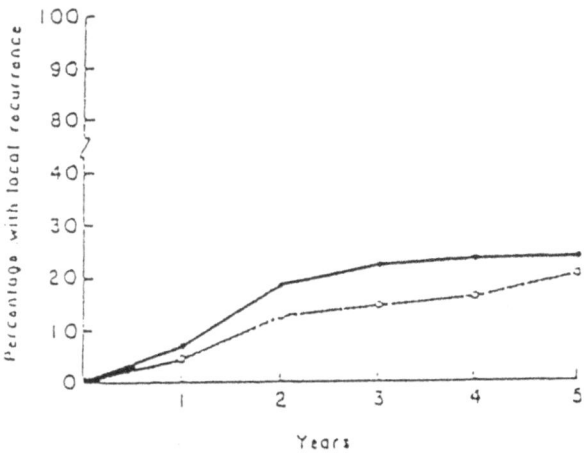

Fig. 14. Cumulative local recurrence rates for anterior restorative resection o---o and abdomino-perineal resection **o---o** (Reproduced from British Journal of Surgery 72:597 by permission of Butterworth & Co)

logical studies have demonstrated that it is not necessary to resect the rectum with a minimum 5cm of distal clearance; 2cm is quite adequate. As a result of these developments, most low rectal cancers can be removed with restoration of intestinal continuity and without the need for a permanent colostomy. An abdomino-perineal excision is now reserved only for very low, locally extensive carcinomas. It has been shown that by applying this philosophy the quality of life for patients is infinitely superior to that after APER, and this has been achieved without survival and recurrence rates being compromised (Figures 13 and 14).

The main problem following low sphincter saving resection for rectal cancer is that some patients suffer frequency of bowel action. This is due to a reduction in compliance of the "neo-rectum". Recently, this problem has been addressed by the construction of a small colonic pouch which increases the storage capacity of the neo-rectum, and seems to reduce the frequency of defaecation. Time will tell, however, whether this becomes a standard modification to the operation.

Local Techniques

If a rectal tumour is small, pathologically not very advanced and accessible, it is feasible to remove it via a transanal approach without the need for a laparotomy. Although there are guidelines as to which tumours can be treated in this way it is impossible to be sure that the associated lymph nodes are not involved and therefore such a local excision cannot guarantee complete excision of malignant tissue. Hence, local excision tends to be reserved for small lesions in patients who are relatively unfit for a major resection.

Contact irradiation or interstitial radiotherapy is an alternative technique to eradicate small rectal cancers, a technique originally pioneered in France. However, the same criticism concerning its failure to eradicate extra rectal malignancy applies.

Other local techniques that are being used, primarily to control symptoms from large rectal tumours in patients unfit for surgery include cryosurgery, electrocautery and Nd Yag laser therapy. The latter is particularly useful for re-establishing the rectal or colonic lumen in patients with obstructing carcinomas. It has the advantage of being able to destroy tissue, and at the same time coagulate it so that haemostasis can be achieved.

Care of Colostomy

Although the aim of surgeons treating colorectal cancer is to eradicate the cancer and at the same time to restore intestinal continuity and continence, there still remains a significant proportion of patients with rectal cancer who will require an abdomino-perineal excision and permanent colostomy. Others, despite having gastrointestinal continuity restored, will need a temporary defunctioning stoma to allow the anastomosis to heal. Consequently, physicians looking after such patients need to have some knowledge of the care of colostomies.

Perhaps the most important part of colostomy management begins before the operation. The patients should be seen by the stoma-therapist and a careful explanation should be given as to what a colostomy entails. Sufficient time should be allowed for the patient to ask questions, and this may require several visits. It is also useful if the patient meets a colostomist who has adapted satisfactorily to the stoma. The stoma-therapist in conjunction with the surgeon should choose a site for the stoma, and the patient should fix an appliance at this site for 24 hours to ensure it is in the ideal place.

Post-operatively, the patients will require encouragement to accept the stoma and will need to be taught how to change the appliance and clean the stoma. Basically, there are two types of management. The "laissez faire" or spontaneous action technique means that the patient keeps an appliance on 24 hours a day and the stoma works when it wishes. With adjustment of diet and judicious use of laxatives or constipating agents some patients manage to obtain a regular, predictable action. The other technique is to use irrigation. This is popular in the USA; approximately 90% of patients use it, whereas in Europe it is less popular. Using an infusion set, the patient instils via a soft cone inserted into the stoma one to one and a half litres of warm tap water. This stimulates the colostomy to work, and after evacuation the appliance is replaced. Ideally, there are no further bowel actions in the next 24 hours, and the patient can sometimes re-

place the appliance with a pad. When successful, the technique gives the patient a degree of confidence and reduces the problem of odour.

In the last decade, great strides have been made in stoma care, and there are now appliances on the market which have significantly reduced the incidence of leakage, odour and skin irritation. Nevertheless, despite these advances, many patients find their colostomies a tremendous burden which affects their social life and pyschological state. Many devices have been tried to ensure that colostomies remain continent; these include an inflatable silastic cuff and the Erlangen magnetic ring. Unfortunately no device has yet been developed which reliably results in continence.

Post-operative Complications of Surgery

The complications of resection for colorectal carcinoma are similar to any major abdominal procedure. They include haemorrhage, wound sepsis, intra-abdominal abscess, deep venous thrombosis and pulmonary embolus, urinary retention and infection, abdominal wound dehiscence, paralytic ileus and mechanical intestinal obstruction. More specific complications depend on the type of procedure performed. Where an anstomosis has been constructed there is a risk of leakage which can cause a pericolic abscess, faecal fistula or frank peritonitis. Whereas anastomotic leakage is uncommon after colonic resection, it still remains a problem for low colorectal or colo-anal anastomoses. For this reason, some surgeons perform a defunctioning stoma at the time of the initial operation to allow healing, and prevent the complications of anastomotic dehiscence. An anastomosis can also contract down to produce a stricture with associated intestinal obstruction. Those patients who undergo abdomino-perineal excision of the rectum may suffer with complications from the perineal wound or colostomy. The perineal wound may become infected and break down, taking months to heal and sometimes leaving a persistent sinus. The colostomy may prolapse, retract or stenose, the skin around it may become excoriated, and a paracolostomy hernia may develop. Excision of the rectum alone, either as part of an APER or a sphincter-saving resection may damage pelvic autonomic nerves, resulting in bladder and sexual dysfunction. After APER, some patients complain of a disturbing sensation, as if the rectum was still in situ, and this is referred to as a "phantom rectum" akin to phantom limb following amputation.

Results of Surgery

Mortality

The operative mortality rate, ie death within the first 30 days following surgery, has gradually decreased and the average rate is approximately 4% in most colorectal units in Europe. There is no significant difference in mortality rates between APER and SSR when used to treat low rectal cancers.

Survival and Local Recurrence

The overall corrected 5-year survival rate following radical resection in most units is approximately 50%. However, survival is influenced by various factors and in particular the pathological stage of the disease at the initial operation. A tumour localised to the bowel wall (Dukes' Stage A) usually does well, whereas one with metastases (Dukes' Stage D) does badly (Figure 15). Similarly, a locally extensive fixed tumour has a worse prognosis than one which is mobile. The lower in the rectum a tumour is situated, the worse the prognosis. Young patients are also reported to have a poor outcome.

Local recurrence rates following surgery for rectal cancer vary considerably from 5% to 25%, the average being 12%. The variation seems to be surgeon related. It has recently been shown that when the surgeon considers that a curative resection for rectal cancer has been performed it is not infrequent that microscopic tumour deposits remain, which lead eventually to local recurrence. This finding perhaps explains to some extent the individual surgeon's variability in recurrence rates. However, even in skilled hands it is inevitable in a proportion of cases that some microscopic deposits will remain. Adjuvant therapy may be of help in the further treatment of such patients if local recurrence is to be prevented.

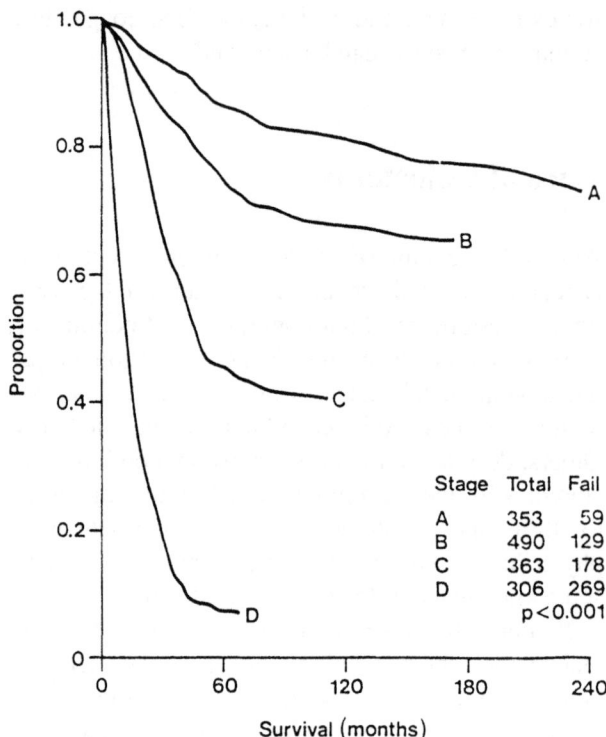

Fig. 15. Survival of patients following resection for colorectal cancer

Stage	Total	Fail
A	353	59
B	490	129
C	363	178
D	306	269
		p<0.001

Adjuvant Radiotherapy and Chemotherapy

The main treatment for colorectal cancer is surgery and attempts to improve disease-free survival by adjuvant therapy have generally met with little success.

Radiotherapy may prolong time without local recurrence of rectal cancer and may even reduce the risk of getting local recurrence. However, the trials which have demonstrated a reduction in the number of local recurrences by adjuvant radiotherapy have all had a rather high rate of local recurrence after surgery alone. The better local control by adjuvant radiotherapy may be associated with increased morbidity, for example intestinal perforation and stricture and intraperitoneal adhesions and, to a lesser degree, damage to the urinary bladder.

Adjuvant radiotherapy should not be used for cancer above the recto-sigmoid juction because of these side effects.

Radiotherapy should not be given to patients with cancers not penetrating the bowel wall (Dukes' A), because they have a very good prognosis from surgery alone. Radiotherapy should not be given to patients with distant spread.

Possible benefit may be obtained in patients with tumours penetrating the bowel wall (Dukes' B) and in patients with regional lymph node metastases (Dukes' C). These are known to have a substantial risk of local recurrence after surgery alone. Radiotherapy may sometimes reduce the size of an inoperable rectal cancer making it possible to remove it by surgery; also, radiotherapy may increase local control of rectal cancers which have not been removed completely according to the pathologist's report.

There are several ways of administrating adjuvant radiotherapy but dosages have to be near maximum tolerable. The sandwich technique takes into account that it may not be possible to exclude tumours not penetrating the bowel wall before surgery. The side effects of radiotherapy may be reduced by giving a boost to the tumour bed intraoperatively after surgical removal of the tumour, but this method is demanding and not feasible in most operating theatres. Possible advantages of preoperative radiotherapy are reduction of tumour size, destruction of tumour cells in lymphatics, vessels and lymph nodes; postoperative radiotherapy makes selection of patients optimal, tumour mass is minimal and surgery is not postponed.

Most studies of adjuvant chemotherapy have shown no effect on survival and risk of local recurrence. Recent data suggest that chemotherapy may prolong disease-free survival. Adjuvant chemotherapy may be used as an infusion of 5-fluouracil into the portal vein. Ongoing trials are evaluating the possible benefits from combining adjuvant radiotherapy and chemotherapy. Chemotherapy includes 5-fluouracil as well as other compounds like nitrosureas and immunotherapeutics. A combination of 5-fluouracil and levamisole may prolong disease-free survival in Dukes' C malignancies, and are now recommended in some countries as a routine, whereas others still evaluate advantages and possible drawbacks in randomised trials of different types of adjuvant chemotherapy.

It may be considered a conservative viewpoint that neither radiotherapy nor chemotherapy should be used as adjuvants to surgery for colorectal cancer. However, more controlled trials are needed before general recommendations can be given.

Pathology of Colorectal Cancer

Colorectal cancers appear in three macroscopic forms which tend to be found in different segments of the large bowel.

1) The ulcerative-infiltrative type shows central excavation with raised, rolled margins. This type is most frequently seen in the rectum and sigmoid.
2) The annular constricting type is also more frequent in the distal colon and produce obstruction.
3) Bulky exophytic tumours are more common in the caecum and ascending colon where they grow intraluminally to a large size before giving rise to symptoms.

Microscopically, the vast majority of malignant neoplasms of the large bowel are adenocarcinomas; other rare tumours include lymphomas, neuroendocrine tumours and small cell anaplastic carcinomas. Most adenocarcinomas are well or moderately differentiated with readily recognisable gland formation and varying degrees of mucin production. Sometimes this latter feature is so marked that the term *mucoid carcinoma* is employed; on rare occasions intra-cellular mucous is conspicuous and gives rise to a *signet-ring cell carcinoma*.

Spread of Carcinoma

1) *Lymphatic spread* results in nodal involvement in a progressive fashion; thefirst nodes to be involved are those closest to the tumour, then spread proceeds centrifugally to involve further nodes in succession and reach the root of the mesentery. The location and number of involved nodes has an effect on prognosis.
2) *Venous spread* Permeation of thin walled veins is a common finding in colorectal cancer. The involved veins can be seen both within the bowel wall and in the surrounding fat. This explains the high frequency of blood borne spread to the liver. Around 25% of patients have overt liver metastases at the time of presentation, and another 20% have "latent" metastases - microscopic tumour deposits that continue to develop after surgery. The finding of extra-mural venous permeation in an operative specimen seems to be related to an increased risk of liver metastases.
3) *Direct spread* Tumour extension occurs by infiltration through the wall and adventitial tissues. Large tumours can spread in this way to involve contiguous structures or organs; rectal cancer into the vagina or prostate, colon cancer into adherent loops of small intestine or the bladder. Tumour may penetrate through the peritoneal membrane and malignant cells disseminate into the cavity giving rise to multiple peritoneal deposits and ascites.

Clinico-Pathological Staging and Prognosis

The extent of spread found pre-operatively and subsequently in a resection specimen, is the principal determinant of prognosis. Thus, the evidence on which prognosis is based can be drawn from clinical and histopathological evidence.

Pre-operative Clinical Assessment

Clinical staging utilises all possible sources of information concerning local and distant spread and allows the most appropriate treatment to be given to the individual patient. Accurate staging permits classification into potentially curative or palliative operations.

1. Assessment of Local Spread (rectal carcinoma)

(I) *Palpation* should be performed in the conscious state. Examination under anaesthesia can be used if this has been inadequate with the patient awake.

(II) *The distance of the lower margin* of the tumour from the anal verge should be determined using a rigid rectoscope.

(III) *Circumferential involvement.* The number and position of quadrants of the bowel circumference which are involved.

(IV) *Fixity.* Tumours should be assessed by palpation as either mobile, tethered (extending through the wall and partially fixed), or fixed to adjacent structures and immobile.

(V) *Scanning techniques.* Whenever available, computerised tomography (CT) should be used to asses the degree of local spread through the wall and to detect the presence of enlarged lymph nodes.

2. Detection of Distant Spread

(I) *Assessment of lung fields.* A chest X-ray should be obtained as routine.

(II) *Detection of liver metastases.* The liver should be scanned in all patients; preferably by CT but failing this, by ultrasound. Serum carcinoembryonic antigen (CEA) should be determined if facilities are available. A high level (50 ng/ml) suggests metastatic disease even if liver imaging is negative.

3. Exclusion of Synchronous Lesions

All patients with a colorectal carcinoma should have the remainder of the large bowel examined. This is best performed by colonoscopy prior to surgery, but if this is not available or is technically impossible (for example, if a stenotic lesion is present) then a double-contrast barium enema should be performed. Where proper pre-operative assessment has not been possible, then synchronous lesions should be sought by intra-operative palpation and (when available) on-table colonoscopy, or by post-operative colonoscopy.

Intra-operative Assessment

During operation the surgeon can confirm the extent of spread and if necessary re-assess the type of operation to be performed. In particular, fixity of the tumour to adjacent structures will modify the operative approach, and the presence of peritoneal metastases, liver metastases and involvement of para-aortic lymph nodes can be confirmed (employing intra-operative frozen section examination when available).

Evidence from Pathological Examination

Pathological staging is an attempt to categorise the extent of disease to give prognostic information following operation. The first priority of the pathologist is to determine whether or not a complete removal has been performed. Even if the resection has been deemed 'potentially curative' on the basis of the pre-operative investigations and intra-operative findings, careful examination of the resection margins - in particular the circumferential margin may reveal microscopic tumour involvement. Having confirmed that the operation is truly 'curative', the pathologist must take a sufficient number of blocks for histology and carefully seek out and examine all the lymph nodes present so that a precise pathological stage can be determined. The principal components of any pathological staging system are the extent of spread through the layers of the bowel wall and the number and location of involved lymph nodes.

The first pathological staging system to be devised was that described by Dukes in which three stages were recognised.

A Carcinoma involving the sub-mucosa or muscularis propria (externa) but not penetrating through it.
B Carcinoma extending through the muscle coat but without lymph node involvement.
C Lymph nodes involved.

This was subsequently modified so that when only nodes in the vicinity of the tumour were involved the case was designated C1 and when nodes at the main vascular tie were involved, C2. When distant metastases (para-aortic lymph nodes, liver etc) were present the case is put into a D category.

The modified Dukes' staging system has been widely employed for many years and gives useful prognostic guidance. Following operation an A case has a 95-99% chance of survival at 5 years, a B case 80-85%, C1 about 50%, C2 about 25%. In considering potentially curative operations however approximately 80% of patients will fall into the B or C1 categories where the prognostic guidance is least clear. In view of this, the TNM (tumour-node-metastasis) classification is preferred in some centres as it gives more detailed information about the depth of invasion and categorises the number of involved lymph nodes so that more stratification can be achieved in the B and C1 groups.

Recently a prognostic system based on extent of spread together with other tumour characteristics has been proposed. This system includes not only depth of invasion and number of involved nodes, but takes into consideration the microscopic character of the invasive margin (whether expansive or infiltrative) and the intensity of the lymphocytic response.

In the future however, it seems likely that purely pathological staging systems will make way for clinico-pathological assessments which may yield the ideal prognostic classification. To this end several major studies are underway to collect both clinical and pathological data which might have a bearing on outcome. The collection of comprehensive clinico-pathological data and correlation with survival will ultimately allow a more precise prognosis to be given and indicate the need for adjuvant therapy in individual cases.

Follow-up After Treatment of Carcinoma

The possible benefit from planned follow-up examinations in patients having had curative surgery for colorectal cancer is a matter of controversy.

No specific tumour markers are available. Measurements of plasma levels of carcinoembryonic antigen (CEA) with intervals of a few months are effective to indicate recurrent disease in some patients, before symptoms develop. However, recurrence is seldom local without accompanying distant spread and it has not been shown in controlled studies that mortality will be reduced and survival prolonged by screening with CEA-measurements for recurrent disease. A large multicentre study in Great Britain addresses this problem. Unfortunately, only a small number of patients with recurrence may be cured but detection of more patients with a small number of liver and/or lung metastases may increase the number having curative surgery for recurrent disease.

The preliminary data from a Danish study suggests that no major benefit can be expected from follow-up. The traditional feeling of safety by joining a follow-up programme may be false and the programme itself is not completely without danger from invasive examinations. In recent years it has been suggested that primary and secondary prevention should carry a higher priority than the expensive follow-up programmes which have not been evaluated according to possible cost-benefit and cost-effectiveness. Referral of patients with symptoms of recurrent cancer to hospital may produce the same results as planned follow-up.

An exception from controversy is evaluation of new treatments for colorectal cancer in controlled trials which makes planned follow-up mandatory.

Also patients with colostomies benefit from follow-up to ensure optimal stoma care.

Another reason for follow-up is the increased risk of developing a new colorectal cancer. Provided that a clean colon was secured by colonoscopy at the time of initial surgery, no new cancer will develop in 5 to 10 years. A safe policy would therefore be to colonoscope with intervals of several years to detect and remove new adenomas which are considered precancerous. In addition, a Hemoccult-II test for bleeding could be done every second year to increase the chance of not overlooking a cancer. A postive test would need a colonoscopy.

Some form of a restricted follow-up may be necessary in patients having had palliative treatment for colorectal cancer, making adjustments necessary in general care and medical treatment of pain and anxiety.

Treatment of Recurrent Disease

Recurrence may be local or distant, local recurrence being more common after surgery for rectal cancer. The commonest site for distant recurrence is in the liver, but occasionally the lungs, bone or skin may be affected. Once diagnosed recurrence is difficult to treat and rarely curable.

The usual treatment for local recurrence is radiotherapy. It is often effective in reducing the size of the lesion and thus alleviates the symptoms, but is rarely curative. Surgery has a limited role and is invariably palliative, being useful to bypass or defunction an obstructing local recurrence. A local recurrence in the pelvis may obstruct one or both ureters, resulting in hydronephrosis and/or renal failure. This can be relieved by nephrostomy or ureteroureteric anastomosis if unilateral. However, at this stage it is probably kindest to treat the symptoms conservatively. Some workers have tried local infusion of 5FUDR into pelvic vessels in order to treat local recurrence but morbidity has been high with little response.

The treatment of multiple liver metastases has also been disappointing. A variety of chemotherapeutic agents have been tried, either singly or in combination which usually include 5-fluorouracill. Although positive response rates have been documented, no prolongation in survival has been shown. A recent innovation has been continual hepatic arterial perfusion of 5FU, using an implantable pump. It remains to be seen whether this technique will prove superior to the results achieved when this drug is administered systemically.

The role of surgery in the treatment of hepatic metastases is primarily to deal with a solitary metastasis. If indeed such a deposit is solitary and is in an operable situation, hepatic resection offers the only hope of cure. Unfortunately, many such lesions, although thought pre-operatively to be solitary, are found at laparotomy to be multiple. However, a small proportion can be resected, and of these patients approximately 25% survive for 5 years.

Despite some optimism for the surgical treatment of solitary hepatic metastases, most patients with hepatic metastases can only be treated palliatively. If pain is a feature and is not controlled adequately by analgesics, the hepatic artery can be ligated and this sometimes improves symptoms. Recently attempts have been made to destroy hepatic metastases by cryosurgery or laser, but such techniques are still at the experimental stage.

Work is progressing on the use of monoclonal antibodies conjugated with cancercidal agents directed to the metastases. The problem with this form of therapy remains the specificity of the antibodies. Another approach has been to use immunotherapy. Both IL2 and lymphokine activated killer (LAK cells) have been used to destroy metastatic colorectal deposits, but unfortunately the response rates are poor.

GPSR Compliance

The European Union's (EU) General Product Safety Regulation (GPSR)
is a set of rules that requires consumer products to be safe and our
obligations to ensure this.

If you have any concerns about our products, you can contact us on
ProductSafety@springernature.com

In case Publisher is established outside the EU, the EU authorized
representative is:

Springer Nature Customer Service Center GmbH
Europaplatz 3
69115 Heidelberg, Germany

Batch number: 09635766

Printed by Printforce, the Netherlands